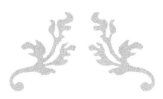

Salad Cookbook

Over 50 Mouth-Watering and Flavorful Salad Recipes to
Prepare For Your Family. Lose Weight, Burn Fat and Reset
Metabolism With Quick and Easy Salad Recipes

Albert Lee

present accurate, up to date, and reliable, complete information. No warranties of any kind are declared or implied. Readers acknowledge that the author is not engaging in the rendering of legal, financial, medical or professional advice. The content within this book has been derived from various sources. Please consult a licensed professional before attempting any techniques outlined in this book.

By reading this document, the reader agrees that under no circumstances is the author responsible for any losses, direct or indirect, which are incurred as a result of the use of information contained within this document, including, but not limited to, errors, omissions, or inaccuracies.

Table of Contents

1. Honey Mustard Potato Salad

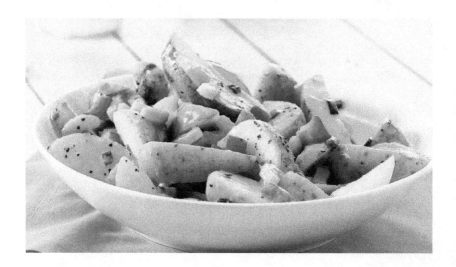

Serving: 4

Prep Time: 55 minutes

INGREDIENTS

- 2 lbs. small red potatoes cut in half

- 4 slices bacon

- 2 tablespoons red wine vinegar

- 1 teaspoon Dijon mustard

- 2 teaspoons honey

- 2 cloves garlic minced

- 1/2 teaspoon sea salt

- 1/4 teaspoon fresh ground pepper

- 1/3 cup olive oil

- 1/4 cup fresh Italian parsley torn

INSTRUCTIONS

- Preheat oven to 375 degrees. Lay bacon on cookie sheet and bake for 7 minutes. Flip and bake for another 7 minutes or until crispy. Move bacon to paper towels.

- Using same cookie sheet with bacon grease on it. Lay potatoes cut side down. Bake for 15 minutes. Flip and bake for another 15 minutes.

- Combine vinegar, Dijon mustard, honey, garlic, salt and pepper. Whisk in olive oil slowly to combine. Coarsely chop bacon. Gently toss potatoes with bacon, dressing and parsley.

Nutritional Contents:

- Calories: 451
- Fat: 29g
- Carbohydrates: 40g
- Protein: 8g

2. Low-Carb Cauliflower 'Potato' Salad

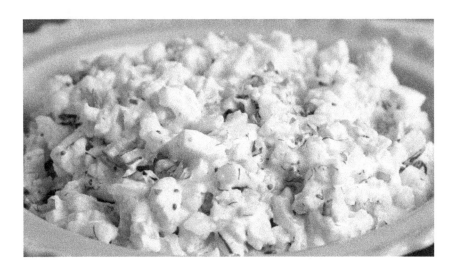

Serving: 5

Prep Time: 50 minutes

Ingredients

- 1 head cauliflower, cored and cut into bite sized pieces

- 3 tablespoons skim milk

- ¼ cup plain, non-fat Greek yogurt

- ¼ cup light mayonnaise

- 2 tablespoons white vinegar

- 1 tablespoon yellow mustard

- 1 teaspoon celery seeds

- ¼ teaspoon salt

- black pepper, to taste

- 4 hard boiled eggs, minus 2 yolks, all diced

- ½ cup diced celery

- 2 green onions, thinly sliced

Instructions

- Bring about 2-3 inches of water to a boil in a large pot and place a steam basket with the cauliflower florets over it. The steam from the water will cook the cauliflower in about 5-7 minutes. Cook until fork-tender.

- You can also steam the cauliflower in the microwave by placing the florets in a large, microwave-safe bowl and adding enough water to just cover the bottom of the bowl. Cover the bowl with plastic wrap and poke some holes in the top. Microwave for 3-4 minutes, or until fork-tender.

- Transfer about ½ cup of the cauliflower to a high-speed blender or food processor with 2-3 tablespoons of skim milk. You just need enough milk to loosen the cauliflower up. Blend into a thick puree, then set aside.

- Transfer the remainder of the hot cauliflower to a colander and run cold water over it to halt the cooking. Set aside to let the water drain.

- In a large mixing bowl, whisk together the yogurt, mayonnaise, vinegar, mustard, celery seeds, salt, and pepper.

- Gently fold in the cooled and drained cauliflower florets, eggs, celery, and green onions.

- Next, fold in the pureed cauliflower, and season with salt and pepper to taste.

- Refrigerate for at least 30 minutes before serving, so the salad gets cold and the flavors meld.

Nutritional Contents:

- Calories: 96
- Fat: 5g
- Carbohydrates: 7g
- Protein: 7g

3. Chickpea Salad

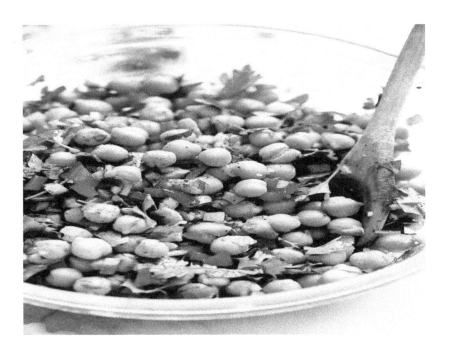

Ingredients

- 1 avocado
- ½ fresh lemon
- 1 can chickpeas drained (19 oz)
- ¼ cup red onion sliced

- 2 cups grape tomatoes sliced
- 2 cups cucumber diced
- ½ cup fresh parsley
- ¾ cup green bell pepper diced

Dressing

- ¼ cup olive oil
- 2 tablespoons red wine vinegar
- ½ teaspoon cumin
- salt & pepper

Instructions

- Cut avocado into cubes and place in bowl. Squeeze the juice from ½ lemon over the avocado and gently stir to combine.
- Add remaining salad ingredients and gently toss to combine.
- Refrigerate at least one hour before serving.

Nutritional Contents:

- Calories: 238
- Fat: 20g
- Carbohydrates: 15g
- Protein: 6g

4. Chicken, Rice, and Black-Bean Salad

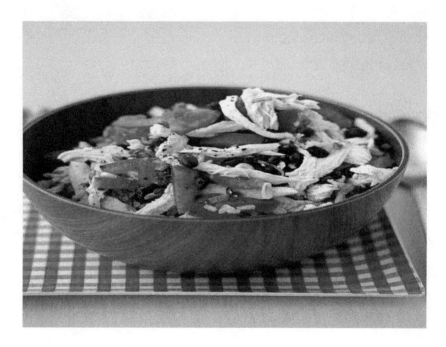

Serving: 4

Prep Time: 60 minutes

Ingredients

- 1 cup brown (or white) rice
- 1 cooked chicken (about 2 1/2 pounds), shredded (about 4 cups)

- 1 can (15 1/2 ounces) black beans, drained and rinsed
- 6 plum tomatoes, quartered lengthwise, seeded, and thinly sliced
- 1 jalapeno chile (seeds and ribs removed for less heat, if desired), minced
- 1/4 cup white-wine vinegar
- 3 tablespoons olive oil
- 1/2 teaspoon ground cumin
- Coarse salt and ground pepper
- 4 scallions, thinly sliced

Directions

- Cook rice according to package instructions. Spread on a baking sheet; refrigerate until cool.
- Place cooled rice in a large bowl; add chicken, beans, tomatoes, scallions, jalapeno, vinegar, oil, and cumin. Season with salt and pepper; toss to combine. Serve immediately, or refrigerate, covered, up to 1 day.

Nutritional Contents:

- Calories: 95
- Fat: 5g
- Carbohydrates: 12g
- Protein: 1g

5. Loaded Veggie Salad Recipe

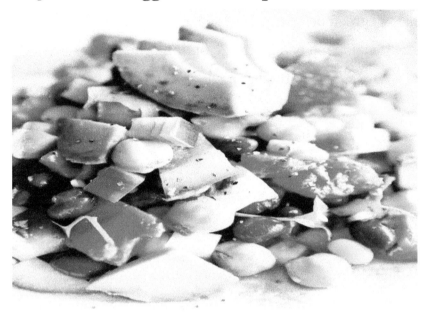

Serving: 8

Prep Time: 20 minutes

Ingredients

- 15 oz black beans rinsed and drained
- 15 oz chickpeas drained (otherwise called garbanzo beans)
- 15 oz diced tomatoes
- 15 oz sweet corn drained
- 4 oz green chilies diced

- 1 red onion chopped
- 1 green bell pepper seeded and chopped
- 1 jalapeno pepper diced, optional
- 1/4 cup cilantro chopped
- 2 limes juiced
- 1/4 cup olive oil
- salt/pepper to taste
- avocado slices for topping

Instructions

- Combine all ingredients (minus avocado) in a large bowl. Mix well.
- Cover and refrigerate until ready to serve. Top with avocado slices just before serving.

Nutritional Contents:

- Calories: 295
- Fat: 5g
- Carbohydrates: 45g
- Protein: 12g

6. Chickpea, Avocado, & Feta Salad

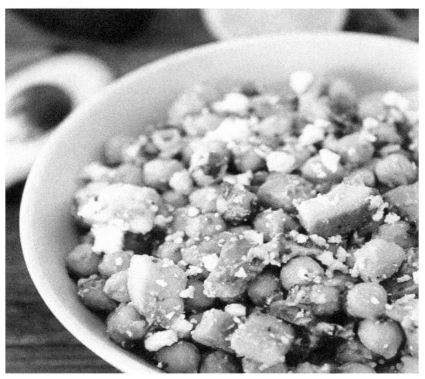

Serving: 4

Prep Time: 10 minutes

Ingredients

- 15 ounces chickpeas, *rinsed and drained*

- 2 avocados, *pitted, and chopped*

- 1/3 cup chopped cilantro

- 2 tablespoons green onion

- 1/3 cup feta cheese

- Juice of 1 lime

- Salt and black pepper, *to taste*

Instructions

- In a medium bowl, combine chickpeas, avocado, cilantro, green onion, feta cheese, and lime juice. Stir until mixed well. Season with salt and pepper. Serve.

Nutritional Contents:

- Calories: 369
- Fat: 20g
- Carbohydrates: 39g
- Protein: 13g

7. Black Bean and Couscous Salad

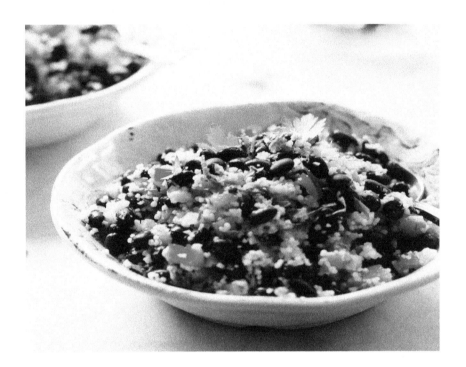

Serving: 4

Prep Time: 10 minutes

Ingredients

- 1 cup uncooked couscous
- 1 ¼ cups chicken broth

- 3 tablespoons extra virgin olive oil
- 2 tablespoons fresh lime juice
- 1 teaspoon red wine vinegar
- ½ teaspoon ground cumin
- 8 green onions, chopped
- 1 red bell pepper, seeded and chopped
- ¼ cup chopped fresh cilantro
- 1 cup frozen corn kernels, thawed
- 2 (15 ounce) cans black beans, drained
- salt and pepper to taste

Directions

- Bring chicken broth to a boil in a 2 quart or larger sauce pan and stir in the couscous. Cover the pot and remove from heat. Let stand for 5 minutes.
- In a large bowl, whisk together the olive oil, lime juice, vinegar and cumin. Add green onions, red pepper, cilantro, corn and beans and toss to coat.
- Fluff the couscous well, breaking up any chunks. Add to the bowl with the vegetables and mix well. Season with salt and pepper to taste and serve at once or refrigerate until ready to serve.

Nutritional Contents:

- Calories: 253
- Fat: 5g
- Carbohydrates: 41g
- Protein: 10g

8. Chickpea Salad with Carrots and Dill

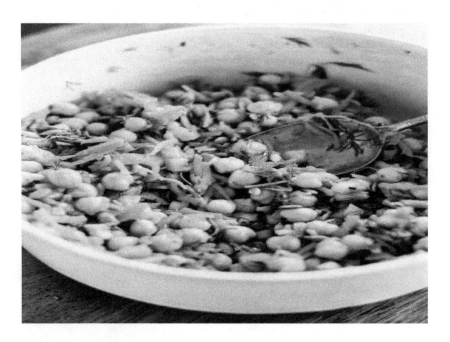

Serving: 4

Prep Time: 20 minutes

INGREDIENTS

- 2 cans chickpeas (15 ounces each), rinsed and drained, or 3 cups cooked chickpeas

- 2 cups grated carrots (about ¾ pound or 5 to 6 medium carrots, peeled and grated on the large holes of a box grater or in a food processor fitted with a grating attachment)

- ⅔ cup chopped celery (about 2 long stalks)

- ½ cup thinly sliced green onions (about 4)

- ½ cup chopped fresh dill leaves (I used one 0.75 ounce package)

- ½ cup pepitas (hulled pumpkin seeds)

- ⅓ cup extra-virgin olive oil

- 2 to 3 tablespoons sherry vinegar

- 1 medium-to-large clove garlic, pressed or minced

- ¼ teaspoon salt

- Freshly ground black pepper

INSTRUCTIONS

1. In a medium serving bowl, combine the chickpeas, carrots, celery, green onions, and dill. Set aside.

2. Toast the pepitas in a small skillet over medium heat, stirring frequently, until they are starting to turn golden and make little popping noises, about 5 minutes. Set aside to cool for a few minutes.

3. To prepare the vinaigrette, in a liquid measuring cup or small bowl, combine the olive oil, 2 tablespoons of the vinegar, garlic, salt, and about ten twists of pepper. Whisk until blended and pour all of the dressing over the chickpea mixture. Add the toasted pepitas to the bowl and stir to combine.

4. Taste, and add additional vinegar (for more zing, I usually add another tablespoon) and/or salt (for more flavor overall, add another pinch). For the best flavor, let the salad marinate for 30 minutes or even overnight in the refrigerator.

Nutritional Contents:

- Calories: 447
- Fat: 28g
- Carbohydrates: 37g
- Protein: 14g

9. Avocado Black Bean Corn Salad

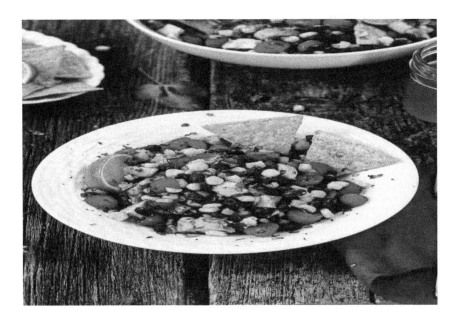

Serving: 6

Prep Time: 20 minutes

Ingredients

Salad

- 2 15 oz cans black beans , drained and rinsed
- 2 avocados , seeded and cubed. (*see note)
- 2 cups corn , fresh or frozen (thawed)

- 2 cups cherry tomatoes , halved
- ½ cup red onion , diced
- ⅓ cup cilantro , rough chopped

Dressing

- ⅓ cup fresh lime juice , more if desired
- 3 tablespoons olive oil , extra virgin
- 1 teaspoon agave (or any sweetener)
- 2 tablespoons fresh cilantro , finely chopped
- ½ teaspoon granulated garlic
- ½ teaspoon chili powder
- 1 teaspoon sea salt , more to taste
- fresh ground pepper , to taste

Cook Mode

- Prevent your screen from going dark
- Instructions
- In a small bowl, whisk the lime juice, olive oil, agave, cilantro, chili powder, granulated garlic, ground pepper, and salt.

- Place all the veggies in a large bowl (except the avocado) and pour the dressing over them. Toss gently to combine well.
- Add the avocado on top and toss gently or just leave them on top. Taste for seasoning and add more if needed.
- Serve immediately with fresh pita bread, tortilla chips or a side of rice. Enjoy!

Nutritional Contents:

- Calories: 291
- Fat: 14g
- Carbohydrates: 33g
- Protein: 7g

10.   Wild Rice Three Bean Salad

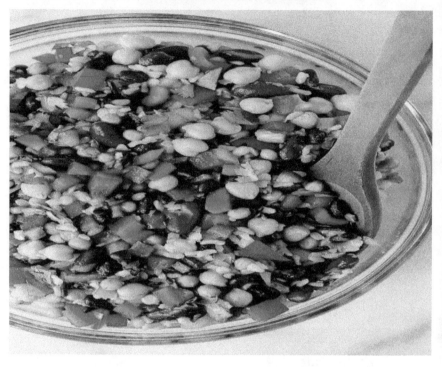

Serving: 8

Prep Time: 10 minutes

Ingredients

- 2 cups cooked wild rice blend cooled

- 15 oz kidney beans rinsed and drained

- 15 oz black beans rinsed and drained

- 15 oz garbanzo beans rinsed and drained

- 1 red bell pepper chopped

- 1/2 red onion diced

- 1/2 cup chopped cilantro

- 1 jalapeno diced

Dressing

- 3 tbsp red wine vinegar

- 2 tbsp extra virgin olive oil

- 4 tbsp sugar

- 1/2 tsp salt

- 1/2 tsp fresh ground black pepper

Instructions

- Combine all salad ingredients in a large bowl.
- Combine dressing ingredients in a mason jar and shake until thoroughly combined.
- Toss dressing with salad.
- Refrigerate for an hour for best flavor but this salad can be served immediately.

Nutritional Contents:

- Calories: 288
- Fat: 5g
- Carbohydrates: 47g
- Protein: 14g

11. Black-Eyed Pea Salad

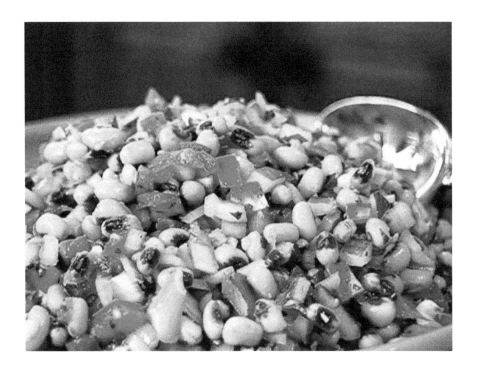

Serving: 4

Prep Time: 10 minutes

Ingredients

- 1 large tomato, diced
- 1/2 medium red onion, finely chopped
- 1 small red bell pepper, finely chopped
- 1 jalapeno, finely chopped
- 2 tablespoons chopped green onions
- 2 tablespoons chopped fresh parsley leaves
- 1/4 cup unseasoned rice wine vinegar
- 1/4 cup canola oil
- 1/2 teaspoon sugar
- Salt and freshly ground black pepper
- Two 15-ounce cans black-eyed peas, drained

Directions

1. Combine the first 6 ingredients in a bowl.

2. In a separate small bowl, whisk together the rice wine vinegar, canola oil, sugar, and salt and pepper.

3. Toss all together with the black-eyed peas and let marinate for at up to 8 hours in the refrigerator before serving.

Nutritional Contents:

- Calories: 95
- Fat: 5g
- Carbohydrates: 12g
- Protein: 1g

12. Healthy Tomato, Basil And Chickpea Salad – Vegan And Gluten-Free

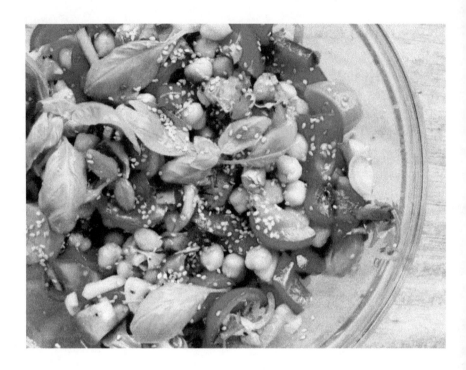

Serving: 4

Prep Time: 10 minutes

INGREDIENTS

- 1 can chickpeas (400g)

- 2 tbsp sesame seeds

- 1 small red pepper

- ½ cup cilantro (chopped)

- 10 basil leaves

- 1 tbsp sesame oil / olive oil

- 2 spring onions

- 1 normal onion (small)

- 1 tsp balsamic vinegar

- 1 tsp nigella seeds (optional)

- 2 big tomatoes

- 1 carrot (optional)

- salt to taste

INSTRUCTIONS

1. Rinse and drain chickpeas and place in a large salad bowl.

2. Chop pepper, cilantro, onions, tomatoes, carrots. Add to chickpeas in the salad bowl.

3. Add sesame oil (olive oil works as well) and balsamic vinegar. Mix everything and add salt if needed.

4. Garnish with basil, sesame seeds, nigella seeds.

Nutritional Contents:

- Calories: 416
- Fat: 21g
- Carbohydrates: 48g
- Protein: 13g

13. Mexican Quinoa Salad with Black Beans, Corn, and Tomatoes

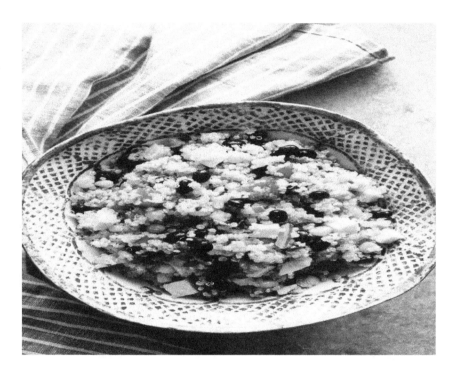

Serving: 4

Prep Time: 10 minutes

Ingredients

- 1 cup uncooked quinoa, well rinsed

- 1/2 teaspoon salt

- 2 cups water

- 1/3 cup diced red onion

- 2 Tbsp lime juice

- 1 15-ounce can black beans, drained and rinsed

- 1 cup frozen corn, defrosted, OR 1 cup of fresh corn, parboiled, drained and cooled (approximately the amount of kernels from one ear of corn)

- 3 medium tomatoes, seeded and cut into chunks

- 5 ounces Queso fresco, Queso Panela, fresh Mozzarella or other mild farmer's cheese, cut into 1/4-inch to 1/2-inch cubes

- 1 jalapeño, seeded and finely chopped

- 1/4 cup chopped cilantro, including tender stems, packed

- 3 Tbsp extra virgin olive oil

Method

- Cook the quinoa:

- Put the rinsed quinoa, salt and water into a pot and bring it to a boil. Cover and simmer gently until the quinoa absorbs all the water, about 10-15 minutes.

- Remove from heat and let sit for 5 minutes. Place into a large bowl and fluff up with a fork to help it cool more quickly.

- Soak onions in lime juice:

- While the quinoa is cooking, prepare the rest of the salad. Soak the red onions in the lime juice and set aside. Soaking the onions in lime juice (or lemon juice or water) helps take the edge off of them.

- Mix the prepped black beans, corn kernels, tomatoes, cheese, jalapeños, cilantro, and oil:

- into a large bowl.

- Add quinoa and onions to bean mixture:

- When the quinoa has cooled, mix it into the bean mixture. Add the red onion and the lime juice and add salt, more oil or lime juice to taste.

- Serve at room temperature.

Nutritional Contents:

- Calories: 95
- Fat: 5g
- Carbohydrates: 12g
- Protein: 1g

14. Zesty Quinoa Salad

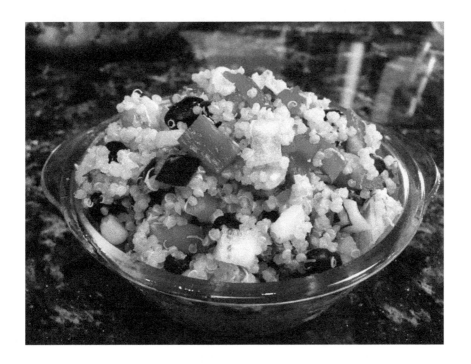

Serving: 6

Prep Time: 30 minutes

Ingredients

- 1 cup quinoa
- 2 cups water

48

- ¼ cup extra-virgin olive oil
- 2 limes, juiced
- 2 teaspoons ground cumin
- 1 teaspoon salt
- ½ teaspoon red pepper flakes, or more to taste
- 1 ½ cups halved cherry tomatoes
- 1 (15 ounce) can black beans, drained and rinsed
- 5 green onions, finely chopped
- ¼ cup chopped fresh cilantro
- salt and ground black pepper to taste

Directions

- Bring quinoa and water to a boil in a saucepan. Reduce heat to medium-low, cover, and simmer until quinoa is tender and water has been absorbed, 10 to 15 minutes. Set aside to cool.
- Whisk olive oil, lime juice, cumin, 1 teaspoon salt, and red pepper flakes together in a bowl.
- Combine quinoa, tomatoes, black beans, and green onions together in a bowl. Pour dressing over quinoa mixture; toss to coat. Stir in cilantro; season with salt and black pepper. Serve immediately or chill in refrigerator.

Nutritional Contents:

- Calories: 95
- Fat: 5g
- Carbohydrates: 12g
- Protein: 1g

15. Costco Quinoa Salad

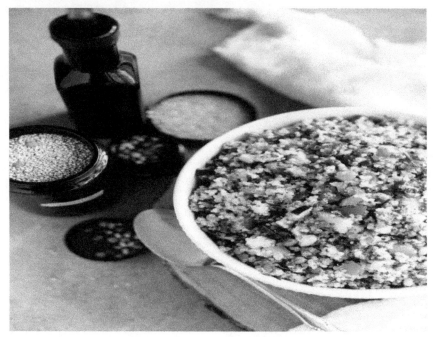

Serving: 4

Prep Time: 35 minutes

INGREDIENTS

- 1 Cup Uncooked Quinoa

- ½ Cup Uncooked Lentils**

- ½ Medium Bell Pepper (Diced)

- ½ Cup Cherry Tomatoes (Diced)

- ½ Medium Cucumber (Diced)

- 1 Cup Kale (Finely Chopped)

- ½ Bunch of Cilantro (Finely Chopped)

- Juice of 1 Lemon

- 3 Tbs. White Wine Vinegar (Or More to Taste)

- Salt + Pepper (To Taste)

INSTRUCTIONS

1. Cook quinoa & lentils according to package instructions; chill for 30 minutes in the refrigerator.

2. While quinoa and lentils are chilling, I like to chop my vegetables.

3. Combine all ingredients in a large mixing bowl.

4. Serve chilled.

Nutritional Contents:

- Calories: 95
- Fat: 5g
- Carbohydrates: 12g
- Protein: 1g

16.Refreshing Quinoa Salad

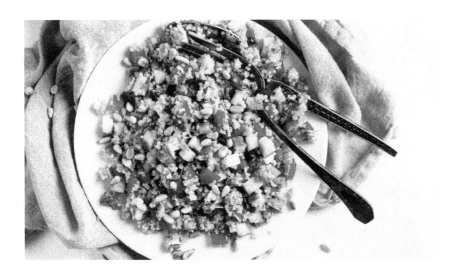

Serving: 12

Prep Time: 10 minutes

Ingredients

- 1 1/2 cups quinoa

- 1 English cucumber, peeled and finely diced (21/2 cups)

- 3 Roma tomatoes, seeded and finely diced (3/4 cup)

- 1/2 small red onion, finely chopped (1/2 cup)

- 1/2 cup chopped fresh parsley

- 1/4 cup olive oil

- 3 Tbs. lemon juice

- 2 tsp. grated lemon zest

Preparation

1. Bring 2 quarts salted water to a boil. Add quinoa, cover, and reduce heat to medium-low. Simmer 12 to 14 minutes, or until quinoa is tender and small "tails" bloom from grains.

2. Preheat oven to 400°F. Spread pine nuts on baking sheet, and toast 3 to 4 minutes, or until lightly browned. Cool, then transfer to large serving bowl.

3. Drain quinoa, and rinse under cold running water. Drain again. Add quinoa to pine nuts, and stir in cucumber, tomatoes, onion, and parsley. Fold in oil, lemon juice, and lemon

zest, and season with salt and pepper, if desired.

Nutritional Contents:

- Calories: 167
- Fat: 10g
- Carbohydrates: 17g
- Protein: 4g

17. Healthy Quinoa Summer Salad

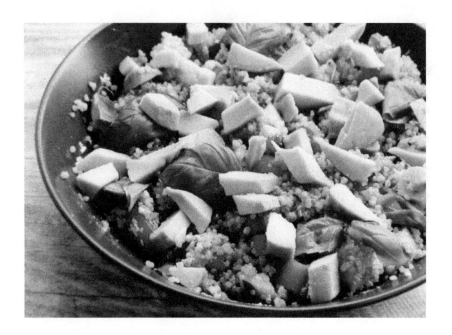

Serving: 4

Prep Time: 10 minutes

INGREDIENTS

- 1 cup cold cooked quinoa

- 1 avocado, seeded, diced

- 1 tbsp lemon juice (about ½ lemon juice)

- 1 small cucumber or ½ of a big cucumber, diced

- 4 spring onions, chopped

- 1 medium tomato, diced

- Optional: some feta cheese

- 1 tbsp vinegar

- 1 tbsp olive oil

- a few basil leaves, chopped

- salt to taste

INSTRUCTIONS

1. Put cooked quinoa, avocado, cucumber, onions, basil and tomato in a large salad bowl.

2. Add lemon juice, vinegar and olive oil and mix everything well. Salt to taste.

3. Optional: add some feta cheese on top.

Nutritional Contents:

- Calories: 95
- Fat: 5g
- Carbohydrates: 12g
- Protein: 1g

18.Cucumber Quinoa Salad

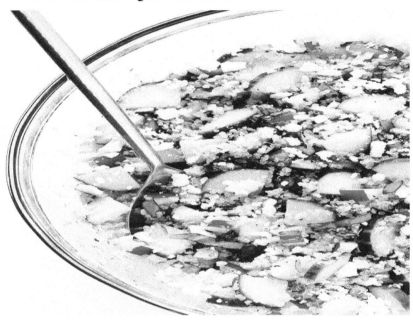

Serving: 4

Prep Time: 10 minutes

INGREDIENTS

CUCUMBER QUINOA SALAD INGREDIENTS:

- 1 English cucumber, diced

- 2 cups chilled* cooked quinoa

- 1/2 cup diced red onion

- 1/2 cup crumbled feta cheese

- 1/3 cup julienned or roughly-chopped fresh basil leaves

- 1 batch Lemony Italian vinaigrette (see below)

LEMONY ITALIAN VINAIGRETTE INGREDIENTS:

- 1/4 cup olive oil

- 2 tablespoons apple cider vinegar or red wine vinegar

- 1 tablespoon fresh lemon juice

- 1/2 teaspoon Italian seasoning, homemade or store-bought

- pinch of salt and black pepper

INSTRUCTIONS

TO MAKE THE CUCUMBER QUINOA SALAD:

1. Toss all ingredients together until combined. Serve immediately.

TO MAKE THE LEMONY ITALIAN VINAIGRETTE:

1. Whisk all ingredients together in a small bowl until combined.

Nutritional Contents:

- Calories: 95
- Fat: 5g
- Carbohydrates: 12g
- Protein: 1g

19. Broccoli Apple Salad

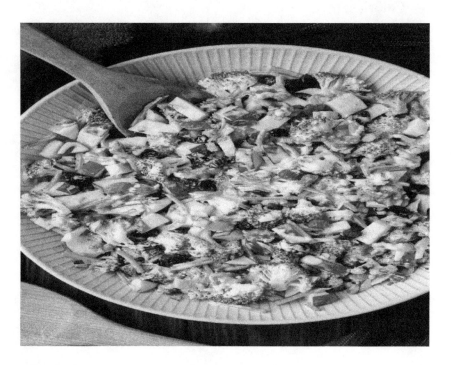

Serving: 8

Prep Time: 20 minutes

Ingredients

- 4 cups small diced broccoli florets

- 2 small gala apples , cored and diced

- 1 cup walnuts

- 1 cup matchstick carrots , roughly chopped

- 1/2 cup golden raisins or dried cranberries

- 1/4 cup chopped red onion

Dressing

- 3/4 cup plain Greek yogurt

- 1/3 cup Hellman's or Best Foods Mayonnaise (full fat)

- 1 1/2 Tbsp apple cider vinegar

- 3 Tbsp honey

- Salt

Instructions

- **For the dressing:**

- In a medium mixing bowl whisk together Greek yogurt, mayonnaise, vinegar, honey and season with salt to taste (about 1/4 tsp). Chill until ready to use.

- **For the salad:**

- In a salad bowl toss together broccoli, apples, walnuts, carrots, raisins or cranberries and red onion. Pour in dressing and toss until evenly coated.

Nutritional Contents:

- Calories: 264
- Fat: 16g
- Carbohydrates: 26g
- Protein: 4g

20.   Broccoli Cauliflower Salad

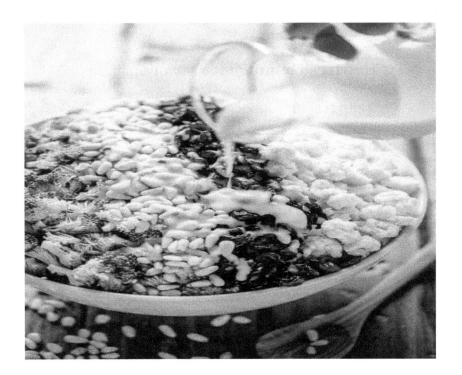

Serving: 4

Prep Time: 10 minutes

Ingredients

- 1 medium broccoli head

- 1 medium cauliflower head

- 3/4 cup dried cranberries craisins

- 1/2 cup sliced almonds or pine nuts toasted on a dry skillet until golden

- 2 Tbsp **honey**

- 2 Tbsp **fresh lemon juice** from 1 small lemon

- 1/2 cup real mayonnaise

Instructions

1. Peel the broccoli stem and chop off the dry base. Chop broccoli into small florets and dice the stem if using.

2. Remove and discard cauliflower core and dice the rest.

3. Toast 1/2 cup almonds on a dry skillet over med/high heat, tossing frequently until fragrant and golden, then add to salad bowl along with 3/4 cup craisins.

4. In a small bowl, whisk together 1/2 cup mayo, 2 Tbsp honey and 2 Tbsp lemon juice. Add dressing to the salad and toss well to combine.

Nutritional Contents:

- Calories: 276
- Fat: 18g
- Carbohydrates: 26g
- Protein: 7g

21.Tortellini Olive Salad

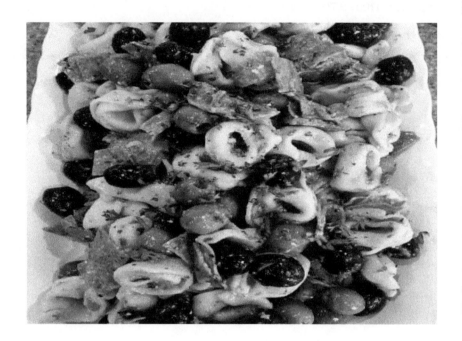

Serving: 8

Prep Time: 30 minutes

Ingredients

- 1 19oz. package frozen cheese tortellini, cooked and drained

- 1 6oz. can of medium size black olives, drained

- 1 7oz jar of manzanilla, green, olives, drained

- 1 14oz. bottle of Bernsteins Cheese Fantastico dressing OR any really good Italian Dressing and 1/4 cup of finely grated Parmesan Cheese. Either will work.

- 1/2 pound hard salami, thinly sliced and cut into bite size pieces OR about 4 slices cut into 1/4 inch thick slices and cubed.

- Chopped parsley and grated Parmesan for garnish

Instructions

1. Follow directions on package of tortellini for cooking pasta al dente. Be sure NOT to over cook the pasta.

2. Cook Pasta and drain.

3. Drain both types of olives.

4. Place the tortellini and olives in a large bowl. Add the diced hard salami.

5. Add 3/4 the bottle, of well shaken, Cheese Fantastico dressing.

6. Stir until all ingredients are well combined. All to chill for 2-3 hours or overnight.

7. Stir just before serving. If needed, add more dressing. Garnish with Parmesan Cheese and chopped Parsley.

8. Serve.

9. Will keep in the refrigerator for 3-4 days.

Nutritional Contents:

- Calories: 470
- Fat: 30g
- Carbohydrates: 28g
- Protein: 22g

22.   Ultimate Greek Chopped Salad

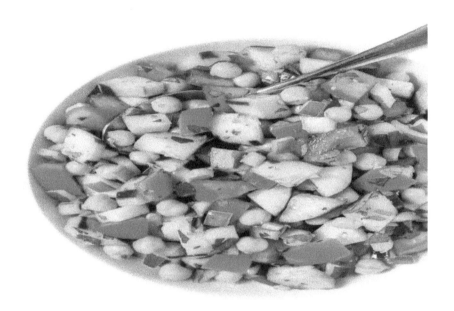

Serving: 6

Prep Time: 15 minutes

INGREDIENTS

- 1 large cucumber (I use hothouse/English)

- 4-5 ripe roma tomatoes (or grape tomatoes)

- 1 large red bell pepper

- 1/2 small red onion

- 15 oz. can garbanzo beans (rinsed and drained)

- *Optional: olives, vegan feta, pepperoncini, fresh herbs*

FOR THE VINEGAR DRESSING:

- 3 Tbsp. red wine vinegar

- 2 tsp. dried oregano

- 1/4 tsp. salt (more/less to taste)

INSTRUCTIONS

- Make the dressing: in a small bowl, combine all ingredients and whisk to combine. Set aside.
- Dice the cucumber, onion, bell pepper and tomatoes (removing any excess liquid from tomatoes).
- Put vegetables and garbanzo beans in a large bowl.
- Add dressing and toss to combine.
- Can eat immediately or refrigerate for at least an hour to let flavors combine. Some dressing will settle on the bottom, so stir before serving.

Nutritional Contents:

- Calories: 95
- Fat: 5g
- Carbohydrates: 12g
- Protein: 1g

23.   Thai Peanut Chicken Crunch Slaw Salad

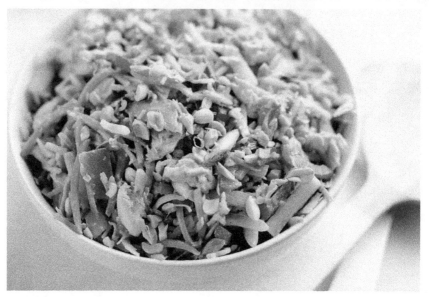

Serving: 6

Prep Time: 20 minutes

INGREDIENTS

- 2 c. coleslaw mix

- 2 c. broccoli slaw

- 1 c. matchstick carrots

- 1 bunch green onions, chopped

- 1/2 red bell pepper, chopped

- 1/2 c. cilantro, chopped

- 1 1/2 c. rotisserie chicken, shredded

- 2 cucumbers, seeded & chopped

- 1 c. thai peanut sauce

- 1 lime, juiced

- 1/2 c. chopped peanuts

INSTRUCTIONS

1. Toss all of the vegetables and chicken in a large bowl. Toss with the Thai Peanut Sauce & lime juice until everything is well coated. Top with peanuts and serve immediately.

Nutritional Contents:

- Calories: 399
- Fat: 23g
- Carbohydrates: 23g
- Protein: 28g

24.   Summer Panzanella

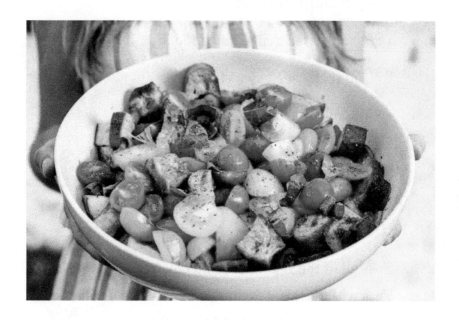

Serving: 6

Prep Time: 25 minutes

INGREDIENTS

- 2 large baguettes, cut into 1-inch cubes
- 1/2 c. extra-virgin olive oil, divided
- 3 tbsp. red wine vinegar
- 1 tsp. honey

- kosher salt
- Freshly ground black pepper
- 1 large, seedless cucumber, roughly chopped
- 2 pt. cherry tomatoes (preferably multi-colored), halved
- 1 red onion, chopped
- 1 clove garlic, minced
- 1 bunch basil, torn

DIRECTIONS

1. Pre-heat a large skillet over medium-high heat.

2. Meanwhile, in a large bowl, toss bread with 1/4 cup olive oil. Add bread to skillet and toast until golden and crisp, about 10 minutes. Drain and set aside to cool.

3. Make dressing: In a small bowl, whisk together red wine vinegar, remaining 1/4 cup olive oil and honey. Season with salt and pepper.

4. To large bowl, add crispy bread, cucumber, tomatoes, onion and garlic. Toss with dressing until evenly coated and season with more salt and pepper.

5. Garnish with basil and serve.

Nutritional Contents:

- Calories: 95
- Fat: 5g
- Carbohydrates: 12g
- Protein: 1g

25. PEA SALAD

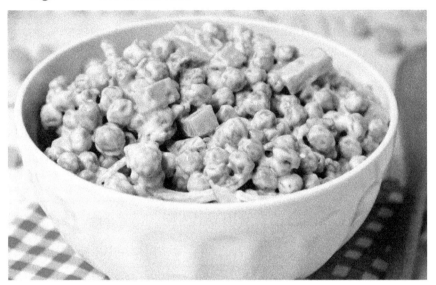

Serving: 4

Prep Time: 10 minutes

INGREDIENTS

- 2-1/2 cups frozen peas, (about 13 ounces)

- 1 cup dry roasted peanuts

- 1 cup chopped celery

- 6 bacon strips, , cooked and crumbled

- 1/4 cup chopped red onion

- 1/2 cup mayonnaise

- 1/4 cup prepared zesty Italian salad dressing

INSTRUCTIONS

1. In a large bowl, combine the first five ingredients. In a small bowl, mix mayonnaise and salad dressing and toss with salad.

2. Refrigerate until serving. If making ahead of time, don't add the bacon. Store separately and toss in before serving to keep crispy.

Nutritional Contents:

- Calories: 95
- Fat: 5g
- Carbohydrates: 12g
- Protein: 1g

26.   MARINATED LENTIL SALAD

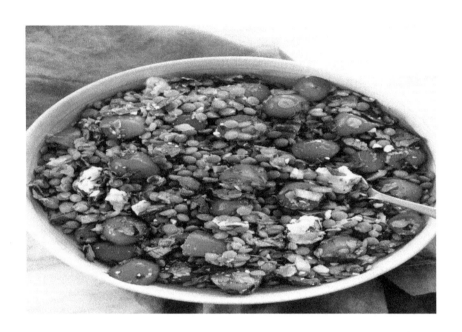

Serving: 6

Prep Time: 30 minutes

INGREDIENTS

LEMON GARLIC DRESSING

- 1 lemon

- 1/4 cup olive oil

- 2 cloves garlic, minced

- 1/2 Tbsp dried oregano

- 1/2 tsp salt

- Freshly Cracked Pepper

SALAD

- 1 cup dry brown lentils

- 1/2 bunch parsley

- 1 pint grape tomatoes

- 1/4 small red onion

- 2 oz feta, crumbled

INSTRUCTIONS

- Cook the lentils according to the package directions. For most brown lentils, bring 3 cups of water to boil in a pot, add the lentils, then continue to boil for 20 minutes, or until the lentils are tender. Drain the lentils in a colander and rinse briefly with cool water until they are cooled.

- While the lentils are cooking, prepare the lemon garlic dressing. Use a microplane, zester, or small-holed cheese grater to remove about 1 Tbsp of the lemon's zest (the thin, yellow, outer layer of the peel). Set the zest aside. Juice the lemon and measure 1/4 cup of the juice to use for the dressing. In a small bowl, whisk together the lemon juice, olive oil, minced garlic, oregano, salt, and some freshly cracked pepper. Set the dressing aside.

- Rinse the parsley well, shake off as much water as possible, then pull the leaves from the stems. Roughly chop the parsley leaves. Cut the grape tomatoes in half. Finely dice the red onion.
- When the lentils are cooked, cooled, and well drained, transfer them to a large bowl. Add the chopped parsley, tomatoes, red onion, crumbled feta, lemon zest, and the prepared dressing. Stir to combine the ingredients and coat everything in dressing.
- Serve immediately, or refrigerate until ready to eat. Always stir the salad just before serving to redistribute the dressing and flavors.

Nutritional Contents:

- Calories:238
- Fat: 11g

- Carbohydrates: 25g
- Protein: 10g

27. SOUTHWEST COUSCOUS SALAD

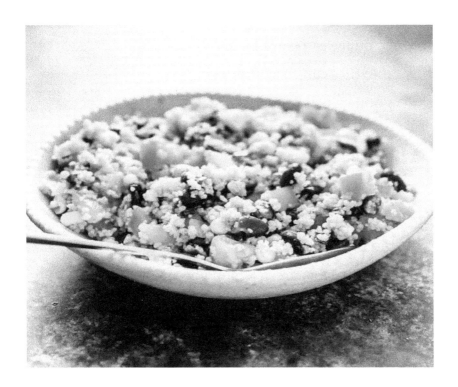

Serving: 6

Prep Time: 30 minutes

INGREDIENTS

- 15-ounce can black beans, drained
- 15-ounce can corn, drained
- 1 orange bell pepper, diced
- 3 roma tomatoes, diced
- 5 scallions, finely sliced
- 1/2 teaspoon ground cayenne (Note 1)
- 1/2 teaspoon garlic powder
- 1/2 teaspoon table salt
- 2 tablespoons fresh lemon juice (Note 2)
- 1/4 cup olive oil

For Cooking Couscous:

- 1 cup couscous (Note 3)
- 1 cup vegetable broth or water
- 1/2 teaspoon table salt

INSTRUCTIONS

- Cook Couscous : Stir together couscous, vegetable broth, and salt in microwave-safe bowl. Microwave for 3 minutes and 30 seconds. Alternatively, cook couscous according to package instructions. Fluff cooked couscous with fork; set aside to cool a bit.

- Combine Salad: Add all ingredients, including cooked couscous, to large mixing bowl. Stir all ingredients together until well-mixed. Serve

Nutritional Contents:

- Calories: 350
- Fat: 11g
- Carbohydrates: 54g
- Protein: 12g

28.　　Guacamole Salad

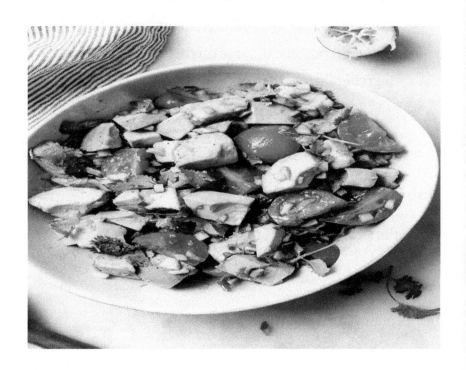

Serving: 4

Prep Time: 10 minutes

INGREDIENTS

- 1/4 c. extra-virgin olive oil
- Juice of 1 lime
- 1/4 tsp. cumin

- kosher salt
- Freshly ground black pepper
- 1 pint cherry tomatoes, halved
- 1/2 c. black beans, drained and rinsed
- 1/2 c. corn
- 1/2 medium red onion, finely chopped
- 1 jalapeno, minced
- 2 ripe avocados, cubed
- 2 tbsp. cilantro, chopped

DIRECTIONS

1. In a small bowl, make dressing: Whisk together olive oil, lime juice, and cumin. Season with salt and pepper. Set aside.

2. In a large bowl, combine remaining ingredients. Toss with dressing until well combined

Nutritional Contents:

- Calories: 95
- Fat: 5g
- Carbohydrates: 12g
- Protein: 1g

29.   Amazing Asian Ramen Salad

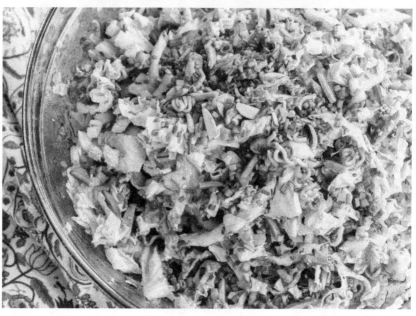

Serving: 8

Prep Time: 2 hour 10 minutes

INGREDIENTS

- 1: 16 ounce bag coleslaw mix
- 1 cup sunflower seeds, de-shelled/shelled/no shells
- 1 cup sliced almonds

- 2: 3 ounce bags ramen*, (any flavor, you won't be using the seasoning packets so it doesn't matter)
- 5 stalks of scallions, sliced
- ¾ cup vegetable oil
- ⅓ cup white vinegar
- ½ cup granulated sugar

INSTRUCTIONS

- In a large bowl, place coleslaw mix, sunflower seeds, sliced almonds, crushed ramen (see note below), and scallions.
- In a large measuring cup, add vegetable oil, vinegar, and sugar. Whisk together. Don't worry if the sugar will not completely dissolve.
- Pour oil mixture over the coleslaw mix and toss everything together with a large spatula until everything is coated well.
- Cover bowl with plastic wrap and chill in refrigerator for at least 2 hours.
- Serve cold or room temperature.

Nutritional Contents:

- Calories: 456
- Fat: 35g
- Carbohydrates: 32g
- Protein: 7g

30.   Carrot Raisin Salad

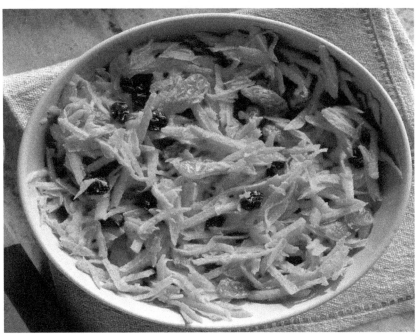

Serving: 4

Prep Time: 10 minutes

Ingredients

- 4 cups shredded carrots

- 3/4 to 1-1/2 cups raisins

- 1/4 cup mayonnaise

- 2 tablespoons sugar

- 2 to 3 tablespoons 2% milk

Directions

- Mix the first 4 ingredients. Stir in enough milk to reach desired consistency. Refrigerate until serving.

Nutritional Contents:

- Calories: 122
- Fat: 5g
- Carbohydrates: 19g
- Protein: 1g

31. TOMATO MOZZARELLA SALAD WITH BALSAMIC REDUCTION

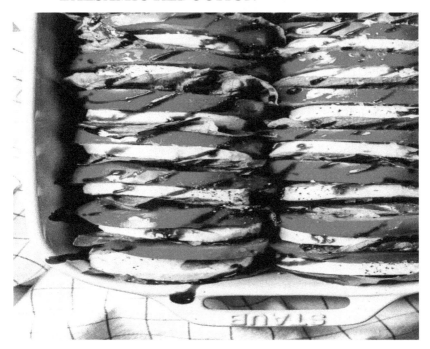

Serving: 8

Prep Time: 20 minutes

INGREDIENTS

- 4–5 hothouse (*beefsteak*) tomatoes, *sliced 1/4-inch thick*

- 2 (16 oz.) logs of fresh mozzarella cheese, *sliced 1/4-inch thick*

- Generous bunch of fresh basil leaves

- Extra-virgin olive oil

- Coarse sea salt and fresh ground black pepper

- Balsamic glaze

INSTRUCTIONS

1. In a casserole type dish (I used 8X11X3) arrange slices of tomatoes, mozzarella, and basil vertically, in an alternating patten until you have created two rows. You may have more rows depending on the size of the dish.

2. Drizzle olive oil over the top of the salad, followed by a drizzle of balsamic reduction.

3. Sprinkle with salt and fresh ground black pepper. Serve immediately.

Nutritional Contents:

- Calories: 375
- Fat: 26g
- Carbohydrates: 12g
- Protein: 20g

32.   Salad On A Stick

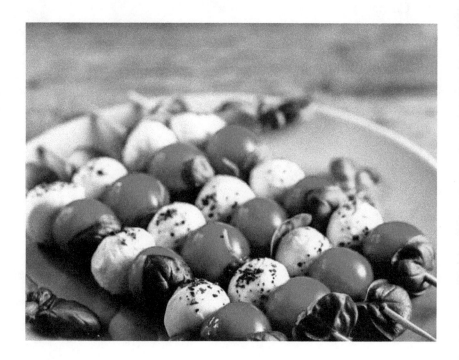

Serving: 4

Prep Time: 10 minutes

Ingredients:

- Iceberg lettuce, cut into chunks about 2-2 1/2 inches
- Cucumber, thinly sliced on a diagonal
- Carrots, thinly sliced on a diagonal
- Grape or Cherry Tomatoes

Directions:

- Thread the carrots, cucumber, lettuce and tomatoes onto long wooden skewers, alternating vegetables. Serve with dressing drizzled over the top or along the side for dipping.

Nutritional Contents:

- Calories: 95
- Fat: 5g
- Carbohydrates: 12g
- Protein: 1g

33.   Mediterranean Couscous Salad

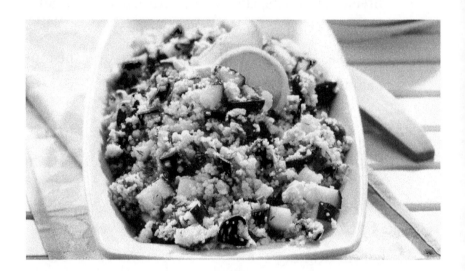

Serving: 8

Prep Time: 20 minutes

Ingredients

- 1 cup Progress chicken broth (from 32-oz carton)
- ¾ cup uncooked couscous
- 1 cup cubed plum (Roma) tomatoes (3 medium)
- 1cup cubed unpeeled cucumber (1 small)
- ½ cup halved pitted kalamata olives
- ¼ cup chopped green onions (about 4 medium)

- ¼ cup chopped fresh or 1 tablespoon dried dill weed
- 2 tablespoons lemon juice
- 2 tablespoons olive or vegetable oil
- 1/8 teaspoon salt
- 2 tablespoons crumbled feta cheese

Direction

- Prevent your screen from going dark while you cook.
- In 2-quart saucepan, heat broth to boiling. Stir in couscous; remove from heat. Cover; let stand 5 minutes.
- In large bowl, place tomatoes, cucumber, olives, onions and dill weed. Stir in couscous.
- In small bowl, beat lemon juice, oil and salt with wire whisk until well blended; pour over vegetable mixture and toss. Cover; refrigerate 1 hour to blend flavors.
- Just before serving, sprinkle with cheese.

Nutritional Contents:

- Calories: 120
- Fat: 5g
- Carbohydrates: 16g
- Protein: 3g

34.   Lemon Orzo Salad with Asparagus and Tomatoes

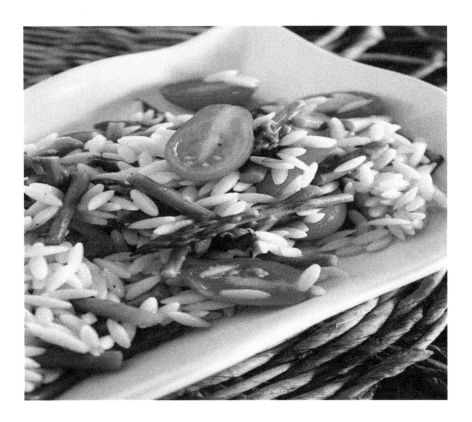

Serving: 6

Prep Time: 60 minutes

Ingredients

- 12 Oz. Orzo
- 1 Bunch Fresh Asparagus
- 1 Pint Grape Or Cherry Tomatoes
- 1 Lemon
- 4 Tbs. Extra Virgin Olive Oil
- 1 Clove Garlic Cloves
- 2 Tbs. Fresh Parsley
- Kosher Salt
- Fresh Ground Pepper
- Grated Parmigiano Reggiano

Direction:

- Bring 2 large pots of water to boil. Add a big pinch of salt in each.
- To one pot, add asparagus and blanch, about 2 to 3 minutes, depending on the thickness of your asparagus. Place blanched asparagus in a bowl of ice water to stop the cooking and keep them green.
- To the second pot, add the orzo. Cook per package instructions. When tender, drain and place in a large bowl. Add blanched asparagus and tomato halves.

- Mix olive oil, lemon zest, lemon juice, garlic, salt and pepper in a small bowl. Stir into orzo and vegetables. Stir in parsley and grated Parmigiano Reggiano.
- This can be served warm, room temperature or cold.

Nutritional Contents:

- Calories: 235
- Fat: 8g
- Carbohydrates: 35g
- Protein: 6g

35. TOMATO BASIL AVOCADO MOZZARELLA SALAD WITH BALSAMIC DRESSING

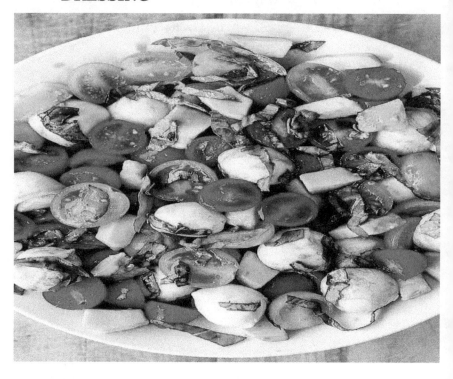

Serving: 6

Prep Time: 30 minutes

Ingredients

Salad ingredients:

- 1/2 pound red grape or cherry tomatoes, halved (2 cups)

- 1/2 pound yellow grape or cherry tomatoes, halved (2 cups)

- 2 avocados , diced

- 8 ounces small fresh mozzarella cheese balls

- 1/2 cup fresh basil , chopped

Dressing ingredients:

- 1/4 cup olive oil

- 1/4 cup balsamic vinegar

- 3 tablespoons honey , warmed

- salt to taste

Instructions

1. In a large bowl, combine all salad ingredients, except Mozzarella cheese balls. That is, combine halved red and yellow grape or cherry tomatoes, diced avocado, chopped basil.

2. In a small bowl, combine all dressing ingredients: whisk olive oil, balsamic vinegar and honey until nice and smooth.

3. Add the salad dressing to the large bowl with salad, sprinkle with a small amount of salt, and toss to combine. Taste and season with more salt, if needed. Add Mozzarella cheese balls on top only at this point - so that they don't brown from the dressing.

Nutritional Contents:

- Calories: 336
- Fat: 27g
- Carbohydrates: 19g
- Protein: 8g

36.　　The World's Best Loaded Chicken Salad Recipe

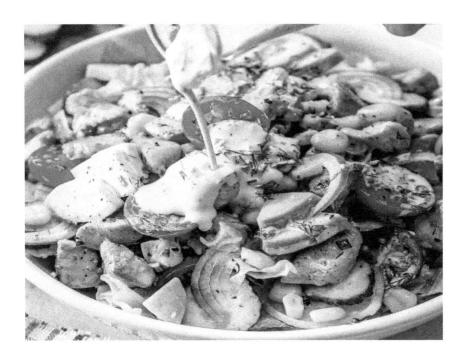

Serving: 6

Prep Time: 20 minutes

INGREDIENTS

- 2 Cups chicken breast shredded or cubed

- ¼ Cup mayonnaise
- ½ Cup sour cream
- 1 Cup celery finely chopped
- 1 Cup sharp cheddar cheese shredded
- ¼ Cup yellow onion finely chopped
- 3 Green onions sliced
- ½ Cup bacon crumbles
- Salt & Pepper

INSTRUCTIONS

- Place the chicken, celery, onions, bacon, and cheese in a large bowl and top with the mayonnaise and sour cream.
- Mix well until everything is evenly coated and distributed throughout.
- Season with salt and pepper to taste. I usually use between ½-1 tsp of each.
- Serve on toast, in an avocado, tomato, in a lettuce wrap, with crackers or your favorite way to eat chicken salad.
- ENJOY!

Nutritional Contents:

- Calories: 114
- Fat: 9g
- Carbohydrates: 3g
- Protein: 8g

37. Best-Ever Chicken Salad

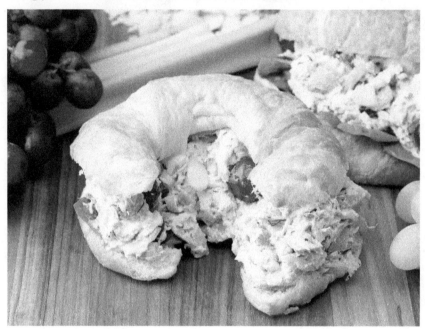

Serving: 10

Prep Time: 1 hour 10 minutes

Ingredients

- 4 lbs chicken parts (bone-in, skin-on thighs and breasts work well) (You'll need about 4 cups)
- 2 tbsp olive oil
- 1 cup grapes seedless, halved (red and green varieties are great)

113

- 1 cup almonds thinly sliced
- 2 stalks celery finely diced
- 3 scallions thinly sliced (white and green parts)
- 2 tbsp dill fresh, chopped
- 1 tbsp parsley fresh, chopped
- 1 cup mayonnaise
- Juice of 1 lemon
- 1 tbsp Dijon mustard
- 1 tsp Kosher salt (start with 1/2 teaspoon, then add more, to taste)
- Freshly ground pepper

Instructions

- Preheat oven to 350°F
- Rub the olive oil all over the chicken pieces and sprinkle with salt and pepper.
- Bake for 45 to 55 minutes, or until internal temp reaches 165°F using an instant-read thermometer.
- Remove the chicken from the oven and let cool. Remove the skin then pull the meat from the bones and roughly chop.
- In a large bowl, mix together the chicken, grapes, almonds, celery, scallions, dill, & parsley.

- In a small-medium bowl, mix together the mayonnaise, lemon, mustard, salt, and pepper.
- Add the mayo/mustard mixture to the chicken mixture and gently stir until well mixed.
- Cover with plastic wrap and refrigerate for at least an hour.
- Serve on a bed of greens with sliced tomatoes and avocado. Or, serve on bread with green leaf lettuce. Add more toppings to your taste!

Nutritional Contents:

- Calories: 273
- Fat: 14g
- Carbohydrates: 7g
- Protein: 4g

38. Mexican Chicken Salad Sandwiches

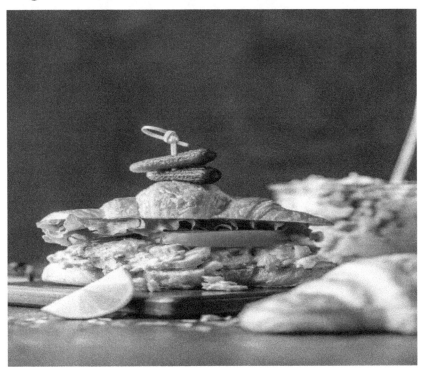

Serving: 4

Prep Time: 10 minutes

Ingredients

- 1 ½ lb cooked shredded chicken breast
- 3/4 cup low fat mayonnaise
- ¼ cup Enchilada Sauce

- ½ ounce Taco Seasoning Click for Homemade Recipe!
- 1 3.5 ounce can Green Chiles
- 1 cup cooked corn
- 1 green pepper diced
- ½ red onion diced
- ¼ cup fresh cilantro chopped
- 1 tablespoon fresh lime juice

Instructions

- Place cooked shredded chicken in a large bowl and add in all other ingredients. Stir to fully combine. Add a bit more mayo if needed for texture.
- Eat in a wrap, on a croissant, on toasted bread, or by itself; the sky is the limit!
- Enjoy

Nutritional Contents:

- Calories: 475
- Fat: 23g
- Carbohydrates: 18g
- Protein: 48g

39.   Jalapeño Popper Chicken Salad

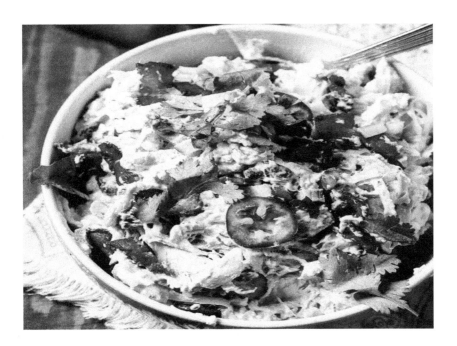

Serving: 8

Prep Time: 60 minutes

Ingredients

- 2 Lbs. Boneless, Skinless Chicken Breast, (pounded to an even thickness)

- Olive Oil

- Salt/Pepper

- 1 teaspoon Garlic Powder

- 1 teaspoon Onion Powder

- 1/2 teaspoon Smoked Paprika

- 1/2 teaspoon Cumin

- 4 Jalapeños, (stems/seeds removed, sliced in half lengthwise)

- 4 ounces Cream Cheese, (softened)

- 1/2 Cup Mayonnaise, (or sub with sour cream)

- 1/2 Cup Chopped Cooked Bacon

- 1/2 Cup Shredded Cheddar Cheese

Instructions

1. Preheat oven to 350°F

2. Place chicken in large baking dish. Coat with olive oil, salt/pepper, garlic powder, onion powder, paprika and cumin. Cover baking dish with foil.

3. Place jalapeños in a separate smaller baking dish. Coat with olive oil, salt and pepper. Cover baking dish with foil.

4. Bake chicken and jalapeños at the same time. Remove jalapeños after 30 minutes. Let cool then chop.

5. Continue to cook chicken until it reaches an internal temp of 165°F (typically 45-60 minutes total, depending on size and thickness) Remove chicken from oven and let cool.

6. Transfer chicken to large bowl and shred with two forks. Add chopped jalapeños, cream cheese, mayonnaise, and bacon. Stir until combined. Salt and pepper to taste then gently stir in shredded cheddar.

7. Serve in wraps, sandwiches, on top of salad, crackers or alone.

Nutritional Contents:

- Calories: 95
- Fat: 5g
- Carbohydrates: 12g
- Protein: 1g

40.   DILL CHICKEN SALAD - LOW CARB, PALEO, WHOLE30

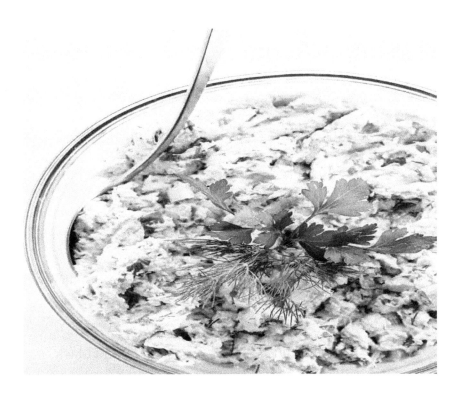

Serving: 8

Prep Time: 10 minutes

INGREDIENTS

SCALE1X2X3X

- 1 pound chicken breast, cooked and cubed

- ½ cup diced celery (one large rib)

- ⅓ cup finely chopped onion

- ¾ cup mayonnaise, more to taste

- 1 tablespoon plus 1 teaspoon Dijon mustard

- 3 tablespoons fresh dill OR 3 teaspoons dried dill

- sea salt and black pepper, to taste

INSTRUCTIONS

1. In a large mixing bowl, combine chicken, celery, onion, mayonnaise, Dijon, dill, sea salt and black pepper. Mix until well combined.

2. Serve on fresh lettuce leaves or just dig right in!

Nutritional Contents:

- Calories: 236
- Fat: 16.5g
- Carbohydrates: 1.5g
- Protein: 12g

41.Avocado Tuna Salad

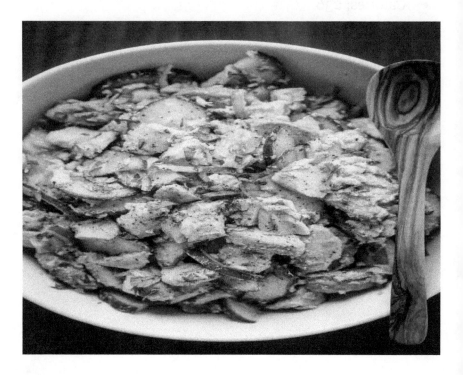

Serving: 6

Prep Time: 10 minutes

Ingredients

- 15 oz tuna in oil, drained and flaked (3 small cans)

- 1 English cucumber sliced

- 2 large or 3 medium avocados peeled, pitted & sliced

- 1 small/medium red onion thinly sliced

- 1/4 cup cilantro (1/2 of a small bunch)

- 2 Tbsp **lemon juice** freshly squeezed

- 2 Tbsp **extra virgin olive oil**

- 1 tsp **sea salt** or to taste

- 1/8 tsp black pepper

Instructions

1. In a large salad bowl, combine: sliced cucumber, sliced avocado, thinly sliced red onion, drained tuna, and 1/4 cup cilantro

2. Drizzle salad ingredients with 2 Tbsp lemon juice, 2 Tbsp olive oil, 1 tsp salt and 1/8 tsp black pepper (or season to taste). Toss to combine and serve.

Nutritional Contents:

- Calories: 304
- Fat: 20g
- Carbohydrates: 9g
- Protein: 22g

42. Panera Tuna Salad Sandwich

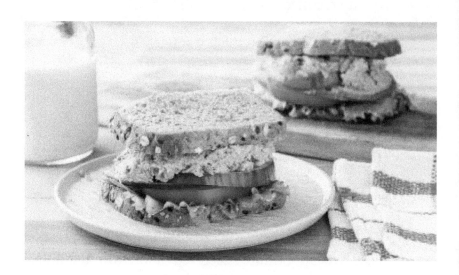

Serving: 4

Prep Time: 10 minutes

Ingredients

- 1 can drained Tuna

- 1 1/2 tsp Mayonnaise

- 1 tsp Sweet Relish

- 3/4 tsp Dijon Mustard

- Salt and Pepper to taste

- Honey Wheat Bread

- Sliced Red Onions

- Sliced Tomatoes

Instructions

1.   Mix tuna, mayonnaise, relish and mustard in a bowl.

2.   Refrigerate for at least 15 minutes.

3.   Serve on honey wheat bread with leaf lettuce, slice red onion and sliced tomato.

Nutritional Contents:

- Calories: 95
- Fat: 5g
- Carbohydrates: 12g
- Protein: 1g

43. White Bean and Tuna Salad

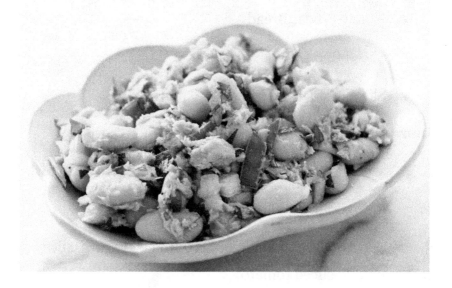

Serving: 4

Prep Time: 10 minutes

Ingredients

- 1 cup of chopped red onions or shallots

- The zest and juice of 1 lemon or 2 limes (can sub a tablespoon or two of cider vinegar)

- 2 five to six ounce cans of tuna packed in olive oil

- 2 15-ounce cans of cannellini or Great Northern white beans, rinsed and drained

- 1/2 cup (loosely packed) of chopped parsley or arugula, or 2 tablespoons thinly sliced mint

- A few splashes of Tabasco sauce, or 1 minced Serrano chile or 1 teaspoon red chile flakes

- 1/2 teaspoon freshly ground black pepper

- Salt and more extra virgin olive oil to taste

Direction

- Sprinkle some of the lemon juice over the chopped onions:

- while you prepare the other ingredients. This will take some of the oniony edge off the onions.

- Combine ingredients in a bowl:

- Drain the oil from the tuna and put the tuna into a large bowl. Add the beans to the tuna and gently stir to combine.

- Add the onions, herbs, black pepper, lemon zest and lemon juice and mix to combine. Add Tabasco or chili to taste.

- If the salad needs more acid, add a little more lemon juice. If the salad seems a little dry, add a little bit of extra virgin olive oil. Add salt to taste.

- Chill before serving:

- This salad will last several days in the fridge, tightly covered.

Nutritional Contents:

- Calories: 195
- Fat: 15g
- Carbohydrates: 12g
- Protein: 16g

44.   Avocado Cucumber Egg Salad

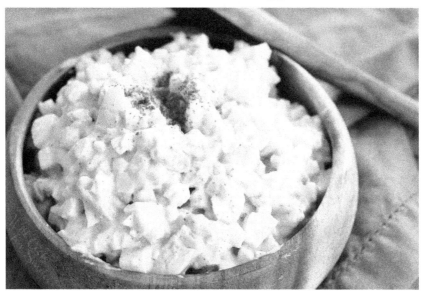

Serving: 4

Prep Time: 10 minutes

Ingredients

- 6 eggs, hard boiled

- 1 cucumber

- 1 lg avocado

- ¼ cup mayo

- ½ tsp paprika

Instructions

1. Hard boiled eggs: bring water to boil in a medium pot (enough to cover the eggs). Add eggs carefully, using a large spoon, so you don't crack the eggs. Cover, boil for about a minute and turn off the heat. Leave the pot on the same burner but with heat turned off. Let eggs sit in the pot for about 20-25 minutes. This method has not failed me yet but you are of course free to use your method of making hard boiled eggs.

2. Peel and dice hard boiled eggs. Add them to a mixing bowl.

3. Peel cucumber, cut it in half lengthwise and scoop out the seeded center, leaving just the outer meat. Dice the cucumber and add it to the eggs.

4. Cut avocado in half. Take out the pit and gentry cut avocado meat lengthwise, then width-wise, not cutting through the avocado skin. Gently peel avocado skin off the meat and add avocado cubes to the mixing bowl.

5. Add paprika, salt and mayo. Very gently, fold the salad, mixing all ingredients until combined.

Nutritional Contents:

- Calories: 95
- Fat: 5g
- Carbohydrates: 12g
- Protein: 1g

45.   Classic Egg Salad

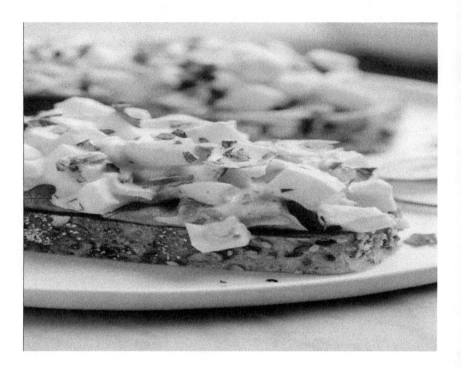

Serving: 8

Prep Time: 4 hour 30 minutes

Ingredients

- 12 hard boiled eggs
- ¼ cup finely chopped red onion
- ¼ finely chopped celery

- ½ cup mayo
- 2 tablespoons yellow mustard
- 1 tablespoon dill pickle relish
- Salt & pepper to taste

Instructions

- Place your eggs in the bottom of a large pot (make sure you use a pot with a lid!), and fill with water. Bring the water to a boil over medium-high heat.
- As soon as it comes to a hard boil, turn off the heat and cover with a lid. then turn off the heat and cover with a lid. Allow to sit, covered, off the heat for 11 minutes.
- While the eggs are sitting and cooking, prepare a large bowl with ice water.
- Place cooked eggs immediately in ice water to cool. Once cooled, crack and peel the eggs. Refrigerate for at least 3 hours until cold.
- When the eggs are cold, finely chop them with a knife or egg slicer and place in a large mixing bowl.
- Add onion, celery, mayo, mustard, relish, and salt and pepper. Stir gently to combine.

- Cover and chill for at least an hour or until ready to serve.

Nutritional Contents:

- Calories: 203
- Fat: 17g
- Carbohydrates: 0.6g
- Protein: 9.3g

46.   Deviled Egg Salad

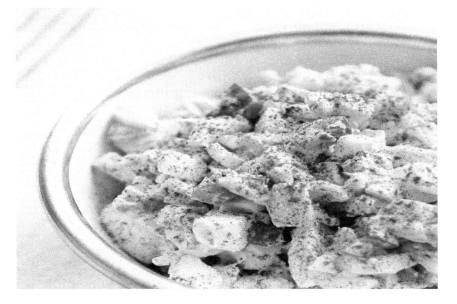

Serving: 4

Prep Time: 25 minutes

Ingredients

- 12 large eggs

- 1/4 cup chopped green onion

- 1/2 cup chopped celery

- 1/2 cup chopped red bell pepper

- 2 tablespoons Dijon mustard

- 1/3 cup mayonnaise

- 1 tablespoon cider, white wine or sherry vinegar

- 1/4 teaspoon Tabasco or other hot sauce (more or less to taste)

- 1/2 teaspoon paprika (more or less to taste)

- 1/2 teaspoon black pepper (more or less to taste)

- 1/4 teaspoon salt (more to taste)

Method

- Hard boil the eggs:

- The easiest way to make hard boiled eggs that are easy to peel is to steam them. Fill a saucepan with 1 inch of water and insert a steamer basket. (If you don't have a steamer basket, that's ok.)

- Bring the water to a boil, gently place the eggs in the steamer basket or directly in the saucepan. Cover the pot. Set your timer for 15 minutes. Remove eggs and set in icy cold water to cool.

- Prep the eggs and veggies:

- Chop the eggs coarsely and put them into a large bowl. Add the green onion, celery, and red bell pepper.

- Make the salad:

- In small bowl, mix together the mayo, mustard, vinegar, and Tabasco. Gently stir the mayo dressing into the bowl with the eggs and vegetables. Add the paprika and salt and black pepper. Adjust seasonings to taste.

- Best served chilled.

Nutritional Contents:

- Calories: 95
- Fat: 5g
- Carbohydrates: 12g
- Protein: 1g

47. The BEST Classic Egg Salad Sandwich Recipe

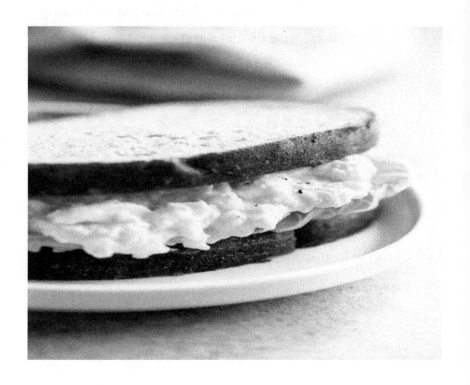

Serving: 4

Prep Time: 10 minutes

Ingredients

- 2 Tablespoons butter, room temperature
- 3 oz cream cheese, room temperature

- 2 Tablespoons celery, minced
- 1 Tablespoon Mayo (or more if desired)
- 1 teaspoon onion, grated
- 1 teaspoon sugar
- 1/2 teaspoon lemon juice
- 1/4 teaspoon salt
- 1/8 teaspoon pepper
- 6 hard boiled eggs, finely chopped or squished with a fork.
- Croissants or Bread
- Paprika (optional)
- Dill Pickle Relish (optional)
- Bacon (optional)

Instructions

- In a medium bowl, cream together butter and cream cheese until smooth.
- Stir in celery, mayo, onion, sugar, lemon juice, salt and pepper until well blended.
- Add eggs and mix well.
- Serve on bread or croissants

- Sprinkle with paprika or add dill pickle relish or bacon if desired.

Nutritional Contents:

- Calories: 82
- Fat: 6g
- Carbohydrates: 5g
- Protein: 2g

48.   Avocado Egg Salad Roll Ups

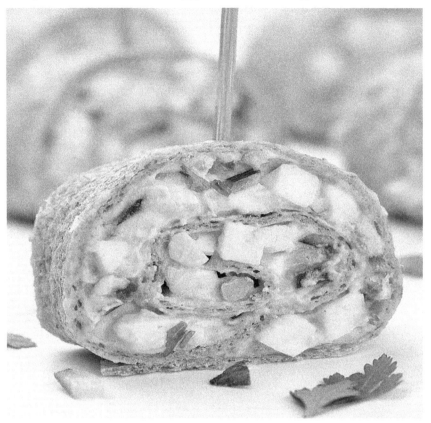

Serving: 4

Prep Time: 10 minutes

Ingredients

- 1 avocado-mashed

- 4–5 hard-boiled eggs chopped in small pieces

- 1 Tablespoon fresh lemon juice

- 2–4 Tablespoons plain Greek yogurt (start with 2 and add more if the salad seems to dry)

- 1 green onion-thinly sliced

- 1 Tablespoon red onion-diced (or more to taste)

- 2 Tablespoons fresh parsley-chopped

- 1/8 teaspoon black pepper

- ¼ teaspoon salt (or more to taste)

- 3–4 whole wheat flour tortillas (8 or 10 inch diameter)

Instructions

1. In a large bowl combine all ingredients (except tortillas) and stir with a wooden spoon until evenly blended.

2. Spread the mixture over tortilla and roll up tightly. Repeat with remaining salad. I had enough filling for 3 10 inch diameter tortillas.

3. Slice with serrated knife into ½- 3/4 inch slices. You can slice them immediately or refrigerate until firm (about 30 mins). It's easier to slice when chilled.

4. Store in the fridge in an airtight container until ready to serve.

Nutritional Contents:

- Calories: 95
- Fat: 5g
- Carbohydrates: 12g
- Protein: 1g

49.   Mediterranean Quinoa Salad

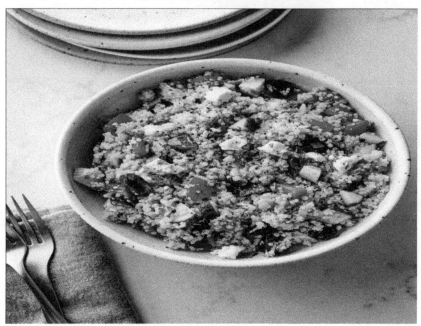

Serving: 12

Prep Time: 22 minutes

Ingredients

- 1 cup quinoa dry
- 1 medium tomato chopped
- 1/2 long English cucumber chopped
- 1 large bell pepper chopped

- 2 large avocado chopped
- 1/4 cup red onion minced
- 1/2 cup parsley or cilantro finely chopped
- 1/2 cup feta cheese crumbled
- 20 Kalamata olives pitted

- 3 tbsp olive oil extra virgin
- 1 lemon or lime juice of
- 1 tbsp cumin ground
- 1/2 tsp salt
- Ground black pepper to taste

Instructions

- Cook quinoa as per package instructions. Or follow my recipes.
- Cook quinoa on the stove: I personally like to cook quinoa with a ratio of 1 cup dry quinoa to 1.5 cups water. Unlike most packages that state 1:2 ratio. Bring to a boil, cook on low for 12 minutes, let stand for 5 minutes and fluff. This way quinoa comes out less mushy.
- Mediterranean Quinoa Salad

- Cook quinoa in Instant Pot: Instant Pot quinoa. It takes 30 seconds of prep and I walk away. Quinoa comes out fluffy and each grain separate after 9 minutes.
- In a large salad bowl, add tomato, cucumber, bell pepper, avocado, onion, cilantro, feta cheese, olives, lime juice, oil, cumin, salt and pepper.
- Mediterranean Quinoa Salad
- Fluff quinoa with a fork and add to the bowl. Stir gently to combine and serve cold or warm.
- Mediterranean Quinoa Salad
- Storing: The beauty of this quinoa cucumber feta salad is that it tastes better with each day. As grains soak up the olive oil, cumin and lemon juices, salad gains more and more flavor. I would say it is good for up to 3 days refrigerated.
- Make ahead: Add all ingredients, except oil, lemon juice, salt, pepper and cumin, to a large salad bowl and do not mix. Cover tightly with plastic wrap and refrigerate for up to 24 hours. When ready to serve, add seasonings skipped previously, then stir and serve.

Nutritional Contents:

- Calories: 348
- Fat: 24g
- Carbohydrates: 8g
- Protein: 29g

50.   Greek Salad

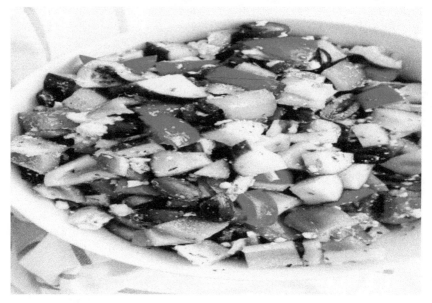

Serving: 4

Prep Time: 10 minutes

Ingredients

- 5 medium-large tomatoes cubed
- 2 large bell peppers cubed
- 1 long English cucumber cubed
- 1/2 cup red onion cubed
- 1 cup pitted Kalamata olives sliced in half
- 1/2 cup feta cheese crumbled

- 1/4 cup extra virgin olive oil
- 2 tbsp red wine vinegar
- 1 tbsp dried oregano
- 1/4 tsp salt
- 1/4 tsp ground black pepper

Instructions

- In a small bowl, combine olive oil, red wine vinegar, oregano, salt and pepper. Whisk and set side.
- In a large bowl, add tomatoes, bell peppers, cucumber, onion, olives and feta cheese.
- Greek Salad Recipe
- Pour dressing on top and stir gently with a large spoon until combined well.
- Greek Salad Recipe
- Best served within 1 hour of combining.
- Greek Salad Recipe
- Make Ahead: Refrigerate salad and dressing separately for up to 2 days, then combine before serving.
- Store: Refrigerate leftovers for up to 12 hours. Salad stays crispy for the evening, after – less.

Nutritional Contents:

- Calories: 143
- Fat: 12g
- Carbohydrates: 8g
- Protein: 3g

CPSIA information can be obtained
at www.ICGtesting.com
Printed in the USA
BVHW011408270721
612866BV00024B/630

9 781802 681703